FREYA GOBER

NATURAL CURES

**The Essential Guide on Natural Cures and Remedies, Discover
How to Cure the Most Common Diseases With Natural Substances**

AF286868

Descrierea CIP a Bibliotecii Naționale a României
FREYA GOBER
  NATURAL CURES. The Essential Guide on Natural Cures and Remedies, Discover How to Cure the Most Common Diseases With Natural Substances / Freya Gober – Bucharest: Editura My Ebook, 2021
  ISBN

FREYA GOBER

NATURAL CURES

**The Essential Guide on Natural Cures and Remedies, Discover
How to Cure the Most Common Diseases With Natural Substances**

My Ebook Publishing House
Bucharest, 2021

INTRODUCTION

Most disease and illness is preventable and curable using natural substances. It's been said that every ailment we face as human beings can be remedied with something in nature. Sometimes it may be bark, leaves, or flowers. Other times it may be an herb, root, or fungi.

This publication is a compilation of tried and true remedies that have been handed down through the ages. As many people are trying to get back to nature and use more raw materials instead of processed poisons, this guide may help you with a cure or remedy for something that ails you.

Age-related Macular Degeneration

It's advisable to eat as many of the following as possible:

- Eggs
- Kale
- Spinach

Allergies

For relief of allergies or colds (stuffy nose, sneezing); try mixing a little diced Garlic with water and drink it.

OR

Mix two grams of garlic oil to one kilogram of water. Drink 20 drops and administer 5 drops in each nostril every four hours.

This also cuts fever and suppresses cough, helps to diminish swelling of the lymph glands, jaundice, pains of muscles or joints, and chronic inflammation of the lungs, associated with these conditions.

A low cholesterol diet and low carbohydrate diet helps to improve Allergy symptoms.

Eat as much of the following as you can:

- Blackberries
- Cranberries
- Garlic
- Kale
- Onions
- Raspberries

To keep your immune system healthy, make sure to get enough lean protein from:

- Seafood
- Tofu

Flaxseeds and flaxseed oil can reduce inflammation. Take 2 tablespoons every day.

Drink 6 to 8 glasses of water a day.

Other recommended foods include:

- Cold-pressed oils

- Fresh vegetables and fruits
- Raw seeds and nuts
- Whole grains

Eliminating foods that cause mucus should be a priority for any allergy suffers. Eliminate the following from your diet:

- Chocolate
- Dairy products
- Eggs
- Fried and processed foods
- Refined flours

Researchers have found if you cook using a gas stove, you are twice as likely to develop breathing problems, like wheezing and shortness of breath associated with asthma.

Alzheimer's Disease

If you want to prevent Alzheimer's, keep yourself active and learning. Avoid sources of aluminum and mercury. Read the labels on antacids, buffered aspirin, deodorants, diarrhea medications, and douches.

A few General Recommendations for Alzheimer's are:

- Acupressure
- Aromatherapy
- Bach flower remedies
- General stress-Reduction Therapies
- Homeopathy
- Massage
- Reflexology
- Regular Exercise – a daily walk…
- Stress reduction
- Wheat Germ

A poor diet, especially one that's high in fat and low in nutrients, can cause a loss of memory, as well as abuse of alcohol or street drugs, inactivity, both physical and mental, medications, heavy-metal poisoning, and more.

Drastically reduce your intake of foods that are high in Cholesterol or saturated fat, they impede blood flow. Avoid sugar and processed foods and stay away from alcohol. Alcohol destroys brain cells.

To help detoxify your body, try a three day juice fast once a month.

Antioxidant vitamins A, C, and E will combat damage from free radicals, which also causes memory loss. A deficiency of the B-complex vitamins can cause memory problems too.

To improve circulation, increase energy levels, and detoxify your body, drink a glass of water every two waking hours.

Some recommended foods are:

- Beans
- Blueberries
- Brewer's yeast
- Eggs
- Fish (mackerel, salmon, and other clean fish, three times weekly)
- Fresh fruits and vegetables
- Nuts
- Oats
- Raisins
- Seeds
- Spinach
- Spirulina
- Strawberries

- Vegetables (raw or lightly cooked)
- Wheat Germ (add to salads, cereals, or juices)
- Whole Grains

Arthritis

An effective diet will go a long way toward controlling arthritis for many people. Eat the following regularly:

- Asparagus
- Broccoli
- Cabbage
- Cauliflower
- Cold water fish (Salmon and mackerel)
- Garlic
- Nuts
- Onion
- Raw pineapple (whole or juiced)
- Raw vegetables
- Seeds (Flaxseeds)
- Tea
- Vegetable oils
- Whole grains

Arthritis Pain

To combat arthritis pain, eat cherries and drink water.

Too much acid in the body causes inflammation which causes pain. Drink a glass of water every two waking hours. Dehydration has been linked to arthritis pain.

Avoid the following:

- Alcohol
- Breads
- Caffeine
- Dairy products
- Eggs
- Fried foods
- Oils
- Pasta
- Pastries
- Red meats
- Refined carbohydrates
- Saturated fats
- Sugar

Rheumatoid Arthritis

Consume the following regularly:

- Asparagus
- Broccoli
- Cabbage
- Canola Oil
- Cauliflower
- Fish (cold water; Salmon and Mackerel)
- Garlic
- Onions
- Pineapple (raw)
- Raw vegetables
- Water
- Whole grains

Asthma

Eat beans and grapefruit on a regular basis.

Airways (Tight)
Eat Beans and Black-eyed peas

Birth Defects

To avoid birth defects, the pregnant mother should eat plenty of:

- Asparagus
- Beans
- Brussels sprouts
- Cauliflower
- Kiwifruit
- Lentils
- Lettuce
- Oranges
- Pasta

- Strawberries
- Wheat Germ

High Blood Pressure

To avoid high blood pressure, you should regularly eat:
- Apricots
- Bananas
- Barley
- Bok Choy
- Celery
- Cereal (Oatmeal, Oat Bran, Whole Wheat)
- Figs
- Fish
- Milk
- Mushrooms
- Nuts
- Oat Straw
- Olive Oil
- Papaya
- Pork

- Potatoes
- Pumpkin
- Squash
- Watermelon
- Yogurt

Low Blood Sugar

Eat three small meals a day, with high-protein snacks in between. A hard boiled egg will lift you out of a mid afternoon slump.

Buerger's Disease

Buerger's Disease is a rare disease of the arties and veins in the arms and legs. It is characterized by a combination of inflammation and clots in the blood vessels, which impairs blood flow. This eventually damages or destroys tissues and may lead to infection and gangrene. This disease usually begins in the hands and feet and may progress to affect larger areas of the limbs.

Virtually everyone diagnosed with this disease smokes; heavy cigarette smokers are most likely to develop Buerger's disease, though it can occur in people who use any form of tobacco, including cigars and chewing tobacco. Quitting all forms of tobacco is the only way to stop Buerger's disease. For those who don't quit, amputation of all or part of a limb may ultimately be necessary.

Increase vitamin E to 1,600 and gradually to 2,400 I.U.s a day, along with lecithin granules and 500 mg. of vitamin C – massage your foot and exercise.

Note: (The International Record of Medicine, July 1951, reports that of 18 patients with Buerger's Disease treated with vitamin E, 17 were cured).

Cancer

The following foods help avoid cancer:
- Apples
- Apricots

- Artichokes
- Avocados
- Bananas
- Beans
- Beef
- Beets
- Bell Peppers
- Blackberries
- Blueberries
- Bok Choy
- Broccoli
- Broccoli sprouts
- Brussels sprouts
- Cabbage
- Canola Oil
- Cantaloupe
- Carrots
- Cauliflower
- Cherries
- Chives
- Corn Cucumbers
- Curry powder

- Fennel
- Figs
- Flaxseeds
- Garlic
- Ginger
- Grapefruit
- Grapes
- Green beans
- Greens
- Horseradish
- Kale
- Kiwifruit
- Lentils
- Mangoes
- Milk
- Mushrooms
- Nectarines
- Nuts
- Okra
- Olive Oil
- Olives
- Onions

- Oranges
- Papaya
- Parsley
- Peaches
- Peanut Butter
- Pears
- Pineapple
- Pomegranates
- Prunes
- Pumpkin
- Quinoa
- Radishes
- Raisins
- Raspberries
- Rosemary
- Seeds
- Shellfish
- Spinach
- Soy
- Squash
- Strawberries
- Sweet Potatoes

- Tea
- Tomatoes
- Vegetable oils
- Whole Wheat Bread
- Wine
- Yogurt

Breast Cancer

Eat grapefruit, oranges, lettuce, and mint on a daily basis.

Please note: Men can also get Breast Cancer and die.

Cervical Cancer

Eat avocadoes, eggplant, and pears.

Colon Cancer

Eat a regular serving of cheese and cranberries.

Prostate Cancer

Eat as much watermelon as you can.

Skin Cancer

Eat the following foods on a regular basis:
- Grains
- Legumes
- Maitake mushrooms
- Nuts
- Organic Juices
- Raw Fruits and Vegetables
- Seeds

Vitamins E and C are believed to lessen the risk of Skin Cancer. Other antioxidants, such as Beta-Carotene, Vitamin A,

Coenzyme Q10, Selenium, Zinc and Bioflavonoids Quercetin and Pycnogenol, could also assist in preventing Skin Cancer.

Antioxidant herbs include Bilberry, Hawthorn, Turmeric, and Ginkgo. Other herbs that aid in the treatment of Skin Cancer are Bloodroot, Pau d'arco, and Chaparral. A cleansing (with a Coffee Enema, Organic Juices and other means), and a highly Alkaline Diet is recommended in the treatment of Skin Cancer.

Things to avoid include pesticides, synthetic hormones and antibiotics, including those used in animal-derived foods. Foods that foster acidity should be minimized, and include caffeine, carbonated beverages, dairy products, liquor, meat, processed foods, and sugar.

Sunburn

If you are subject to sunburn, eat a high beta-carotene diet. Vitamins E and C help to prevent sunburn, which can lead to Skin Cancer.

Collagen and Skin – Take vitamin C to fight Collagen and to help keep your skin looking fresh and young instead of dry and saggy. Take Niacin for nice skin, and vitamin A for added protection, trim the fat to help prevent skin cancer and beta carotene beats harmful sun rays that harm the skin.

Tumors

Applying poultices of Comfrey to tumors (such as tumors in the nose and mouth) has been known to make the swelling and the tumor, gradually disappear, but you should seek immediate medical care first; self-treatment is not recommended unless your doctor approves.

Note: Both green and black teas have proven health benefits. Green tea is clearly the healthier choice. In Japan, where green tea is a part of a typical daily diet, they have twice the smoking rate of the U.S., but only half the rate of lung cancer. Green tea and tea extract contain strong antioxidants that can help stop the formation and development of some tumors.

Skin

For more beautiful and healthier skin, you need antioxidants, Vitamin D, Omega-3s, Coenzyme Q10, and 1,500 mg of Glucosamine included in your daily diet. Ensure that you eat plenty of:

- Berries
- Broccoli
- Cantaloupe
- Fish (cod, mackerel, salmon, sardines, and tilapia)
- Flaxseed and Flaxseed Oil
- Fortified Eggs
- Leafy Greens

Leslie Baumann, M.D. says, "Foods that are bad for your skin include refined sugar that causes the skin to age more quickly, making your skin dryer, thinner, and more prone to wrinkles, dairy foods may exacerbate acne, excessive alcohol may worsen Rosacea, and can lead to broken capillaries, and spicy foods can also aggravate Rosacea".

To ensure soft, supple skin, eat the following:

- Apricots
- Cantaloupe
- Carrots
- Winter Squash

Hives

Stop the itch by soaking in Colloidal Oatmeal, (Aveeno)

Poison Ivy

To relieve the itch, soak a washcloth in cold milk and make a compress for your itchy skin.

Cardiovascular Function and Circulation

Eat the following regularly:

- Grapes
- Cayenne
- Oranges
- Soybean lecithin

High Cholesterol

Choose from the following and eat them regularly. To avoid becoming bored of the same food, rotate what you eat on a daily or weekly basis.

- Apples
- Apricots
- Artichokes
- Avocados
- Barley
- Beans

- Blackberries
- Canola Oil
- Cereal (Oat Bran, Oatmeal, Whole Wheat)
- Chicken
- Chives
- Figs
- Garlic
- Grapefruit
- Lentils
- Margarine
- Oranges
- Parsley
- Peanut Butter
- Pears
- Peas
- Pork
- Prunes
- Raspberries
- Soy
- Tomatoes
- Watermelon
- Wheat Germ

Colds and Upper Respiratory Problems

Colds

Garlic works faster than vitamin C for curing colds. Keep a clove of garlic in your mouth and your cold will disappear within a few hours, or at most half a day, in many cases. It will not burn unless you chew it. Just score it with your teeth, every so often to release a little juice.

If garlic is too strong, try Rocambole or Sand leeks. A sore throat can be stopped in minutes and it even works for sore throat symptoms of diphtheria. Garlic has a curative effect on chronic diseases in the upper respiratory organs, absorbing the poisons. This is also true for "chronic inflammation of the tonsils, salivary glands and neighboring lymph glands, empyema of the maxillary sinus, severe pharyngitis and laryngitis" and other conditions. Garlic gives permanent, not just temporary relief. You can also consume:

- Bell Peppers
- Cauliflower
- Chicken

- Garlic
- Shellfish
- Tea

Stuffy Nose

Eat the following:
- Chilies
- Chicken soup (with fresh garlic and ground cayenne pepper; inhale the fumes while you eat the soup).
- Curry Powder
- Horseradish

Upper Respiratory Infection

Eat chicken soup.

Constipation

Eat the following:

- Barley
- Lentils
- Oat Straw
- Strawberries
- Whetberries

As a bedtime snack, eat a sliced pear mixed with a couple of prunes and a teaspoon of bran.

And drink extra water.

Regularity

Eat the following regularly:
- Apples
- Artichokes
- Barley
- Beets
- Blackberries
- Cereal (Oat Bran, Oatmeal, Whole Wheat)
- Flaxseeds
- Figs

- Lentils
- Lettuce
- Nectarines
- Pears
- Peas
- Prunes
- Quinoa
- Raisins
- Raspberries
- Strawberries
- Wheatberries
- Whole Wheat Bread

Depression

Eat the following:
- Asparagus
- Avocadoes
- Bananas
- Beans (Black Beans and Navy Beans)
- Canola Oil

- Chestnuts
- Chicken
- Eggs (Hard Boiled)
- Flaxseeds
- Fish – Cod, Salmon, Flounder, Halibut, Mackerel, Tuna, Blue fish, Herring, Striped Bass
- Fish Oil
- Grapefruit
- Kale
- Legumes
- Lemons
- Liver
- Mushrooms
- Nuts
- Olive Oil
- Pumpkin Seeds
- Prune Juice
- Quinoa
- Sweet Potatoes
- Spinach
- Sunflower Seeds
- Turkey

- Turmeric
- Walnuts
- Watermelon
- Wheat Germ
- Whole Wheat Bread

Stay Happy

Eat the following:
- Chilies
- Chocolate
- Garlic
- Pasta
- Potatoes
- Prunes

Diabetes

The most important therapy for Type 2 Diabetes is a healthful diet to help regulate your levels of sugar and reduce your risk of complications, such as cardiovascular disease. A diet that's high in fiber with vegetable, nuts, seeds, and whole grains, is optimal. Ground flaxseeds should be consumed daily. Consume 1 tablespoon with each meal or ¼ cup daily. Drink 10 oz. of water per tablespoon of flaxseed. Protein drinks that have low sugar levels can be consumed as well.

Diabetics can benefit from increasing the relative amount of protein in the diet. Do not go longer than three hours without eating. Chromium deficiency has been linked to diabetes, so eat lots of Brewers yeast, cheese, garlic, onions, soy products, wheat germ, and whole grains. Focus on foods with a low glycemic load value.

- Apples
- Barley
- Beans
- Beets
- Berries
- Brewers yeast
- Brown Rice
- Cereal
- Cheese
- Chicken

- Cinnamon
- Curry Powder
- Fish
- Garlic
- Grapes
- Kamut
- Kiwifruit
- Legumes
- Nuts
- Oats
- Oat Bran
- Onions
- Peas
- Plums
- Quinoa
- Seeds
- Soy products
- Spelt
- Sweet Potatoes
- Turkey
- Wheatberries
- Wheat germ

- Whole grains
- Whole Grain Bread
- Whole Grain Cereals
- Whole Grain Pastas
- Whole Wheat Bread
- Wine

Diabetics should avoid white, refined bread, as it spikes your blood sugar. Stay away from simple sugars such as, candies, cookies, sodas, and other sweets. Avoid cow's milk and eliminate alcohol and caffeine from your diet. Cut back on your consumption of saturated fat, found in red meat and dairy precuts, as these have been shown to increase the risk of diabetes and heart disease.

Exercise to avoid Type 2 or Noninsulin-dependent diabetes.

Over 16 million people in the U.S. are afflicted with some form of diabetes, but only half of them know about it. The onset of diabetes can be so gradual that sometimes, a person could be suffering permanent damage from the disease for years before realizing that they have it.

Symptoms of diabetes include an increase in thirst and the need to urinate more. You may lose weight despite feeling hungry more often. You might also notice tingling or complete loss of feeling in your hands or feet or blurred vision. If you have any of these symptoms, see your doctor.

Here's a simple test that helps determine diabetes risk. Answer True or False to the following questions. The more you answer True, the more likely you are to be a candidate for diabetes.

- I am over 40.
- I get little or no exercise during a normal day.
- I am 20% or more overweight.
- I have a parent with diabetes.
- I have a sister or brother with diabetes.
- I am a woman who has had a baby weighing more than 9 pounds at birth.

Insulin Sensitivity

Eat the following regularly:
- Cereal
- Oat Bran
- Oatmeal
- Whole Wheat

Diverticulosis

Eat Wheatberries.

Ears and Hearing problems

For an earache, wrap some Garlic in some gauze and place it in the outer ear canal.

Hearing Can be Improved Up to 90%

You can use this method to help bring back hearing. Press the tip of the third, or ring finger, for about 5 minutes, several times a day. Press the finger on the left hand for the left ear, and right hand for the right ear. Pressure on the joints of this finger may also help. This is said to help improve up to 90% of hearing loss in cases of deafness due to thickening of the ear membrane, ear noises, and ringing in the ears, but everyone can obtain some benefit.

Some foods and a low cholesterol and low carbohydrate count may ease your hearing problems, says Dr. J.T. Spencer, Jr.

of Charleston, W. VA. Sudden deafness requires immediate medical attention, due to its many possible causes such as certain types of infection, a blood clot, poor circulation or other causes.

Hardening of the arteries can lead to an insufficient supply of blood to the inner ear, causing sudden deafness; says Dr. O. Erick Hallberg in the Journal of American Medical Association, November 30, 1957. The continuing use of nicotinic acid, a B vitamin, in high dosages seems to be most beneficial both for its artery widening effect and for its apparent tendency to reduce the blood cholesterol level.

Foods that contain the B vitamins include:

- Brewer's Yeast
- Liver
- Wheat Germ

A low fat diet includes:

- Eggs
- Fresh Fruits
- Fresh Vegetables
- Gravy
- Lean Meats

- No Butter
- Processed cheeses
- Starches

While deafness caused from an insufficient blood supply is fairly consistant, with ringing in the ears and dizziness, other types of deafness may come and go. It is not likely to affect both ears at the same time.

Using lots of soybean lecithin every day can help to reduce or stop the ringing in the ears and clear hearing.

Using garlic oil by puncturing a garlic oil capsule and pouring it into the ear and stopping it with a little cotton can help to relieve earaches.

Some people have had good results in helping to clear up bad hearing and ringing in the ears by using a drop of onion juice in the ears about every week to ten days to help maintain good results.

Chewing gum that contains a natural sweetener called xylitol has been found to help prevent tooth decay and ear infection. Xylitol prevents bacteria form attaching itself to the back of your mouth, where it can later enter your ear and set off an infection.

Note: Too much noise can cause hearing loss, but vitamin A can protect your hearing.

Eating Disorders

For, eating disorders don't diet, instead, cut caffeine, divide single meals into several smaller ones, record everything you eat, schedule your meals and snacks, eat a nutritious, sugar-free diet, include complex carbohydrates with each meal, and take a Zinc supplement to zap eating disorders.

Weight Control

Eat the following:
- Artichokes
- Avocados
- Beans
- Blackberries
- Celery
- Chicken
- Chives

- Cucumbers
- Fennel
- Figs
- Garlic
- Ginger
- Green Beans
- Milk
- Nuts
- Peanut Butter
- Radishes
- Rosemary
- Shellfish
- Tea
- Wheatberries
- Yogurt

Exercise

Without exercise, even the best weight loss plan won't give you the results you're hoping for. Exercise helps you lose weight faster and keeps it off longer.

Eyes

The use of alcohol and tobacco is very bad for your eyesight.

Garlic contains the thiamin-boosting ingredient which increases the body's absorption of B-1 (thiamin) tenfold. Garlic has a curative effect on eye catarrh and inflammation of the lachrymal (tear) duct.

The common herb Comfrey used as a poultice or tea drinks, seems to possess extraordinary healing powers. Doctors have used its medicinal extract, allantoin, in cases of stubborn ulcers, burns, and open wounds, with spectacular results, even burns to the eyes.

Many cases of near blindness have been helped by nerve massage. For eye weakness, massage the pads of the base of the second and third fingers on both hands, left hand for left eye, and right hand for right eye. Pressure on the ends of these fingers can relieve eye strain in a few minutes. To stop watering eyes, massage the webs between these fingers.

Cataracts

Consume the following:
- Kiwifruit
- Onions
- Spinach
- Tea

Cataracts are a loss of transparency of the crystalline lens of the eye. In the most common form, vision becomes blurry, like a frosted glass window, and there is profuse tearing and irritation.

It has several forms, but in general, the lens is hardened and is a deep brown, green, gray or milky. In some cases, it only affects part of the eye.

Using 15 mg of B-2 (tablet form) daily and nothing else, cures almost 100% of the reported cases for Cataracts. These results were reported by Dr. Sydenstricker of the University of Georgia.

Foods containing vitamin B-2:

- Beans
- Beets
- Broccoli
- Brewer's Yeast
- Calf Liver
- Chicken
- Nuts
- Peanuts
- Raw Collards
- Salmon
- Turnip Tops
- Wheat germ

The lack of vitamin C and Calcium are often associated with Cataracts. Others advise the use of vitamins A, D, E, dessicated liver, sunflower seed meal, organex, and protein, in addition to vitamin C and B-2 for Cataracts. This combination also helped with mental and physical health.

In Eye, Ear, Nose and Throat Monthly (volume 31), a doctor says that his method of preventing or correcting cataracts is to give his patients a special diet which includes the tops of vegetables with a pint of milk and two eggs daily, with vitamins C and A and chlorophyll tablets.

Foods rich in calcium (all contain roughly 200mg. per serving) include:

- Common Beans
- Beet Greens
- Dandelion greens
- Mustard greens
- Parsley
- Turnip greens
- Watercress

Corneal Ulcers

Corneal Ulcers are relieved by using 1500mg. of vitamin C according to The British Medical Journal, November 18, 1950.

Glaucoma

It is extremely important not to attempt to treat glaucoma yourself by dietary measures, without your doctor's approval. This disease has several forms and needs to be treated precisely. Glaucoma patients who self-treat run the risk of blindness. Glaucoma can literally wipe out your vision overnight.

To help reduce the pressure of the eye that causes Glaucoma symptoms, one woman used 2,000 to 3,000 mg. of vitamin C with rose hips plus 150 mg. of Rutin twice a day for three months. The pressure in her eyes returned to normal. Others report the same results.

Eating three carrots a day boiled in about a quart of water. Drink all of the water and use no seasoning.

Take 3 tablespoons of raw liquid lecithin daily. It cleans out the bloodstream and can help to greatly improve eye sight.

Cut out coffee and take Vitamins A, B, C, E, and bone meal. Vitamin C lowers eye pressure.

Macular degeneration

A low fat diet helps control Macular degeneration, which deprives the individual of a the ability to see straight ahead. In most cases, it's due to a blockage or leak in the tiny blood vessels which interlace the macula, a round light-sensitive spot at the center of the retina.

Night Blindness

Eat Spinach.

Seeing Spots

Floaters can be relieved with B vitamins. If you should ever experience dark black spots, you should have it checked out, it could be something serious.

Vision

Foods that help near and far sightedness:

Vitamin A is essential to good vision. A mild deficiency makes it difficult to see at night. A more severe form results in headaches from bright light. Burning, itching and gritty sensation under the eyelids may develop. In advanced stages, pus and ulcers may form and you may see dark spots called scotomata. To remedy this, eat foods that are rich in Vitamin A, like:

- Beet greens
- Dandelion leaves
- Chard (cooked)

Other foods good for vision include:

- Bell Peppers
- Berries
- Broccoli
- Cabbage
- Cantaloupe
- Carrots
- Corn
- Eggs
- Garlic
- Grapes
- Greens – Mustard greens, turnip greens
- Kale
- Kiwifruit
- Mangoes
- Nectarines

- Onions
- Papaya
- Parsley
- Peaches
- Plums
- Pumpkin
- Spinach
- Squash
- Sunflower Seeds
- Tea
- Watercress
- Sunflower seeds have been found to relieve farsightness, eye strain, aches and pain, and extreme light sensitivity. They contain 50 units of vitamin A per 100 grams, and are also rich in B complex vitamins, iron and calcium. Take three teaspoons of Sunflower seed kernels daily.

Puffy Eyes

For puffy allergy eyes, place a cucumber slice on each eye for a couple of minutes. The cucumber slices cause blood vessels to constrict, which could help to reduce the puffiness.

Vision Development in Infants

Feed your baby fish, and flaxseeds

Gallstones

Eat oranges.

Gout

Consume the following:
- Berries
- Cherries (drink a glass of cherry juice every day)
- Fish (Cod, Halibut, Salmon, and Sardines; they reduce inflammation)
- Flaxseeds (add to juices, salads, or fruit plates, or use the oil as a salad dressing)
- Nuts
- Raw fruits and vegetables
- Seeds
- Soy products
- Whole grains

Drink a glass of water every two waking hours. This should be your minimum consumption. Rich foods aggravate gout pain. You must not drink alcohol in any form.

Foods to avoid in your diet should include:

- Anchovies
- Asparagus
- Brewer's Yeast
- Broths
- Bouillon
- Consommé
- Dried Beans
- Eggs
- Fish
- Gravies
- Herring
- Lentils
- Meats
- Mushrooms
- Peas
- Poultry
- Red meat
- Sardines

- Shellfish
- Spinach and Rhubarb (cooked)
- Sweetbreads

To reduce the risk of Heart Attack

Eat the following:

Brown Rice and other whole grains

Soybean lecithin (every day) will help to cleans out fat-encrusted veins and arteries.

Irregular Heartbeat

Eat the following:
- Fish
- Watermelon

Heartburn

Eat Curry powder.

Heart Disease

Include the following in your regular diet:
- Apples
- Artichokes
- Asparagus
- Avocados
- Bananas
- Barley
- Beans
- Beef
- Beets
- Bell Peppers
- Blackberries
- Blueberries
- Broccoli
- Brown Rice
- Brussels sprouts
- Cabbage
- Canola Oil
- Cauliflower

- Cereal (Oat Bran, Oatmeal, Whole Wheat)
- Cherries
- Chicken
- Chilies
- Chives
- Chocolate
- Cinnamon
- Cranberries
- Cucumbers
- Eggs
- Figs
- Fish
- Flaxseeds
- Garlic
- Grapes
- Green Beans
- Greens
- Horseradish
- Kale
- Kiwifruit
- Lentils
- Lettuce

- Mangoes
- Margarine
- Nuts
- Olive Oil
- Olives
- Onions
- Oranges
- Papaya
- Parsley
- Pasta
- Peaches
- Peanut Butter
- Pears
- Pineapple
- Pomegranates
- Pork
- Prunes
- Pumpkin
- Quinoa
- Raisins
- Raspberries
- Rosemary

- Seeds (Pumpkin, Sesame, Sunflower)
- Shellfish
- Soy
- Squash
- Strawberries
- Sweet Potatoes
- Tea
- Tomatoes
- Turkey
- Vegetable Oils
- Watermelon
- Wheatberries
- Wheat Germ
- Whole Wheat Bread
- Wine

Hemorrhoids

It is estimated that 50 to 75 % of Americans will suffer from Hemorrhoids at least once. Nearly 1/3 of the population has an ongoing problem with this often painful condition.

To remedy the problem:

- Eat in a relaxed atmosphere, breathing and chewing food thoroughly.
- Eat smaller, more frequent meals and avoid overeating at one sitting.
- You should eat 5 – 9 servings of fruit and vegetables every day.
- You should drink 8 or more glasses of water every day.

Eat or increase polyunsaturated fats and eat a high-fiber diet which includes:

- Alfalfa sprouts
- Almonds
- Apricots
- Unpeeled Apples
- Beans
- Berries

- Cayenne
- Cold-water fish
- Dark berries
- Dried beans
- Figs
- Flaxmeal (1 heaping tsp. in 8 oz. of apple juice, followed with an additional 8 oz. of water.)
- Ginger Root
- Green leafy vegetables
- Nuts
- Kale
- Kefir
- Kelp
- Oat Straw
- Peas
- Prunes
- Raw Fruits and Raw Root Vegetables… (Jicama, Turnip Roots, Radishes, and Carrots).
- Sauerkraut
- Seeds (Dried Pumpkin and Sunflower Seed)
- Stewed or Soaked Prunes… (one to three times a day).
- Unsweetened Live Yogurt

- Wheatberries
- Wheat germ
- Whole Grains
- Whole grain Bread

Eliminate refined foods such as:
- Alcohol
- Caffeine
- Dairy products
- Spicy foods
- Sugars

Decrease your intake of animal products and saturated fats
You need the following vitamins:
- Vitamin C (1,000 mg two to three times per day)
- Vitamin E (400 to 800 IU per day)
- Vitamin K will stop or prevent bleeding.

Do not use laxatives and get regular exercise.

For temporary relief of pain and itching, use any of the following as a topical lotion:
- Calendula gel

- Cocoa butter
- Olive oil
- Zinc oxide

Hypoglycemia

Eat eggs

Hypothyroidism – Underactive Thyroid

Natural thyroid hormone is more effective than the synthetic type, but it is more difficult to obtain. Under proper circumstances, Vitamins A, C, B complex, B12, E, coenzyme Q10, magnesium, manganese, zinc, selenium, iodine, amino acid tyrosine, DHEA, and melatonin may be beneficial.

Aerobic exercise may help to correct a low-thyroid condition.

It is never advisable to drink tap water. Most tap water is full of fluorine and chlorine, two chemicals that inhibit your ability to absorb iodine. Ensure that you eat plenty of:

- Cocoanut oil

- Flaxseeds
- Fish
- Sea Salt
- Sea Vegetables (Dulse, Kelp, Kombu, Nori, and Wakame)
- Walnuts

Avoid the following foods unless they are cooked. Cooking the vegetables inactivates the goitrogens found in the following foods, so that they are safe to eat for someone with low thyroid:

- Broccoli
- Brussels sprouts
- Cabbage
- Cauliflower
- Kale
- Soy

Kidneys and Kidney Stones

Many people with kidney stones suffer from dehydration. While you have the kidney stone, drink 2 ½ to 3 quarts of water every day. Once the stone has passed, resume a normal daily dose of 1 glass every two waking hours. Hydration is the single most important tactic in the treatment and prevention of kidney stones. If you must eat animal products, stick to lean, high-quality sources of white meat. A magnesium deficiency has been linked to recurring kidney stones. Ensure you eat plenty of:

- Almonds
- Apples
- Bananas
- Beans
- Celery
- Fish
- Fresh – raw vegetables
- Green leafy vegetables
- Kelp
- Kidney Beans
- Lemon juice (mixed with a little hot water)
- Nuts
- Oat and Wheat Bran (daily)
- Orange juice
- Parsley
- Pumpkin seed (1/4 cup daily)
- Seeds
- Soybeans

- Watermelon
- Whole grains

Eliminate foods that contain high amounts of oxalic acid from your diet. By far, the worst offenders are:

- Alcohol
- Almonds
- Blueberries
- Blackberries
- Beets
- Caffeine
- Celery
- Concord Grapes
- Cocoa
- Collards
- Dairy Products (milk, cheese, ice cream)
- Eggplant
- Grapefruit (studies show that grapefruit increases the risk of kidney stones)
- Parsley
- Peanuts
- Red meat

- Rhubarb
- Refined Sugar (soft drinks that contain phosphoric acid)
- Salt (reduce the intake)
- Spinach
- Strawberries
- Summer squash
- Sweet Potatoes
- Tomatoes

Osteoporosis

Eat the following regularly:
- Almonds
- Black beans
- Broccoli
- Calcium-enriched rice milk or soymilk
- Collard Greens
- Fish
- Flaxseeds
- Green leafy vegetables (except spinach)
- Kale
- Lentils
- Miso
- Molasses
- Milk
- Nuts
- Oysters
- Romaine Lettuce
- Sardines (with bones)

- Sea vegetables (Agar, Nori, Kombu, Tempeh, and Wakame,)
- Sesame seeds
- Shellfish
- Spinach
- Tofu
- Unsweetened cultured yogurt
- Walnuts
- Yogurt

A high salt intake has been linked to Osteoporosis.

Women who drank more than 14 glasses of milk a week had 45% more hip fractures then women who consumed 1 glass a week or less. Calcium from cow's milk is not well absorbed. You should avoid sugar, refined grains, and soda pops. You should reduce your intake of red meat which may contribute to bone loss in some individuals.

For Osteoporosis, you need the following intake…

Calcium – 500 to 600 mg twice daily in divided doses.

Magnesium – 250 to 300 mg twice daily in divided doses.

Vitamin D – 800 to 1,200 IU daily if you have osteoporosis and 400 IU daily if you are supplementing vitamin D for prevention.

Vitamin K1 is the form of vitamin K found in plants that is important for bone formation. Take 2 to 10 mg daily and up to 500 mcg daily for preventative purposes.

Ipriflavone – 600 mg with food. Have your lymphocyte, a type of white blood cell_ levels monitored by your doctor when using this supplement.

Essential fatty acids – 4 grams of fish oil daily, along with 3,000 mg of evening primrose oil.

Strontium – 680 mg daily.

To maintain and build healthy bones

Eat the following:
- Almonds
- Asparagus
- Basil
- Bok Choy
- Broccoli

- Brussels sprouts
- Cabbage
- Cantaloupe
- Carrots
- Celery
- Cheese
- Cherries
- Eggs
- Fish
- Flaxseeds
- Garlic
- Greens
- Kale
- Milk
- Miso
- Nuts
- Okra
- Onions
- Oranges
- Parsley
- Pork
- Potatoes

- Rhubarb
- Seeds
- Shellfish
- Soy
- Squash
- Tea
- Tofu
- Walnuts
- Water (drink a glass of water every two waking hours)
- Wheat Germ
- Wine
- Yogurt

Foods high in sulfur will help repair cartilage and bones.

Restless Leg Syndrome

Restless leg syndrome is often associated with iron deficiency anemia. Eating iron-rich foods like red meat, nuts, and beans may help, but too much iron can be harmful, so have your iron levels checked by your doctor and don't take iron supplements without a doctor's advice.

Sinusitis

During an acute infection, eat lightly and drink one glass of water every two waking hours, drink plenty of herbal teas, vegetable juices, and broths.

For a powerful sinus drainage remedy, eat a small spoonful of crushed horseradish mixed with lemon juice. You may want to be near a sink or have a towel handy after taking this potent combination.

If you must take an antibiotic for a sinus infection, be sure to consume a nondairy source of friendly bacteria, such as kefir or sauerkraut.

To alleviate Sinusitis, consume the following:

- Alcohol
- Cayenne
- Chicken soup (especially with lots of vegetables)
- Cold-pressed oils
- Flaxseeds (will reduce inflammation; add to cereals or salads)
- Flaxseed oil (will reduce inflammation; take 1 tsp of oil every day)
- Fresh Fruits and Vegetables
- Garlic

- Horseradish
- Kefir
- Onions
- Peaches
- Raw Nuts and Seeds
- Salt (severely restrict your intake)
- Sauerkraut
- Watermelon
- Whole Grains
- Oranges
- Garlic

Foods to avoid:

- Chocolate
- Dairy products
- Eggs
- Flours (Refined)
- Fruit Juices
- Fried and processed foods
- Sugar

To relieve a sinus headache and floaters from your eyes, take two grams of vitamin C every hour for about 16 hours. The number of hours depends on how bad your symptoms are.

74

Darrhea, Indigestion, Gastritis, Nausea and, Stomachache ailments

Diarrhea

Eat the following:
- Applesauce
- Artichokes
- Bananas
- Rice
- Toast
- Yogurt

Indigestion

Eat the following:
- Artichoke
- Curry Powder
- Ginger
- Mangoes
- Mint

- Pineapple
- Yogurt

Gastritis

Eat Oat Straw.

Morning Sickness and Nausea

Eat grapes and watermelon

Motion Sickness

Eat the following:
- Candied Ginger
- Ginger tea
- Olives

Stomachache

Eat dried Blueberries and Mangoes.

Eat a few tablespoons of dried blueberries. It has been reported that blueberries inhibit the ability of bacteria to stick to the inside of your body, which reduces the chance of a nasty infection in the lining of your stomach. Fresh or frozen berries may aggravate tummy troubles.

Upset Stomach

Eat Mangoes and Mint

Food Poisoning

The most important thing is to keep hydrated by drinking two cups of liquid every waking hour. Try broths, electrolyte drinks, diluted fruit and vegetable juices, and water.

Foods easy to digest are soups, broths, and steamed vegetables. You should stay away from dairy products, fats, and oils. Avoid sugar, caffeine, and alcohol. Once you begin to feel better, these foods tend to taste especially good:

- Apples
- Bananas
- Brown Rice
- Carrots
- Cooked fruits
- Vegetables
- Soups

Stroke

If you're at a high risk for a stroke, especially with high blood pressure, which increases your odds, start eating at least five fruits and vegetables a day, especially citrus fruit and vegetables from the cabbage family, like Brussels sprouts. You can also consume:

- Apples
- Bananas
- Brussels sprouts
- Cabbage
- Canola Oil
- Cauliflower
- Eggs
- Figs
- Fish
- Ginger
- Grapefruit
- Kiwifruit
- Nuts
- Onions
- Oranges
- Pumpkin
- Quinoa
- Squash
- Tea
- Watermelon

- Wheat Germ
- Wine

Gums, Mouth Sores, Teeth, Throat, and Tongue

Bleeding Gums

For bleeding gums, take 20 mg. of zinc and 500 mg. of vitamin C daily.

Eat a diet of natural foods and lots of vitamin C to help fight the deterioration of bones and infections of the gums, etc.

Canker Sores

Eat yogurt

To dry up and heal canker sores, hold a wet tea bag in your mouth over the canker sore; adjusting the bag from time to time for comfort, but keep it over the sore for at least 10 minutes. Dandelion tea may also heal cankers and prevent their return.

For early treatment of canker sores, punch a hold in a vitamin E capsule and squeeze the gel directly on the ulcers as soon as they appear. This can be repeated from time to time until the sores are healed. A good gargle can work wonders too.

Cold Sores

Outbreaks of cold sores can be triggered by stress, which weakens the immune system. According to researchers, one of the best things you can do to keep away these painful sores is to relax.

Teeth

Eat garlic and oranges. Garlic makes loose teeth take root again and removes tartar.

Tooth Decay

Eat cheese, drink tea, brush your teeth and visit a dentist.

Sore Throat

While this in not a cure - it has been used to relieve the horrible pains of throat cancer.

Violet Leaf Tea, used as a drink, mouthwash or gargle. Use of this common tea is not permitted without a doctor's approval and is no substitute for qualified medical care.

To make the Violet Leaf Tea; use 2 ½ oz of fresh leaves of the Prince of Whales Violet, the kind that grows wild or in you Grandmothers garden, in a pint of boiling water. Don't use the general herricks variety (the large florist violets sold in nurseries as Viola Odorata).

Tongue Soreness and Burning Remedy

To relieve soreness of the tongue, take large doses of Vitamin C.

To relieve a burning tongue, take a liver supplement along with vitamin B-12 and riboflavin.

Bad Breath

Chew on a fennel seeds or munch on a sprig of parsley.

Ulcers

Eat the following:

- Basil
- Chilies
- Cinnamon
- Tea

Urinary Tract Infection

Eat blueberries and cranberries

Varicose Leg Ulcers

Make a poultice using Comfrey. Put several big leaves through a juicer, dilute them, put the pulp on some gauze, and use this poultice just once a day for about six weeks.

For Diabetic's Varicose Vein; increase vitamin E to 3,000 I.U.s and vitamin C to 2,000 mg daily.

Warts

Take 500 mg of Olive leaf Extract twice daily. Apply one drop of Garlic Oil to the wart(s) twice daily for 4 weeks. Garlic Oil has antiviral properties. Take 200 mcg of Selenium daily. A Selenium deficiency makes it easier for viruses to replicate. Take 400 IU of Vitamin E daily. Vitamin E is important for immune function and to combat viral infections.

Other Health Issues and Notes…

- To cool a hot head from the heat, put a chilled lettuce leaf under your cap.
- Research shows that foods cooked in cast-iron skillets are higher in iron.
- Quick egg substitute for cooking: Mix 1 Tblsp. of milled flaxseeds with 3 Tblsp. of water and let stand for a minute or two. Add to the recipe in place of an egg.
- Fight stress with Ginseng.

Note:

If you are using a salt substitute to reduce your salt intake, use it sparingly. Many salt substitutes contain sodium, just smaller amounts. If you shake it too much, you may be getting the same amount of sodium as you would get in salt. Some salt substitutes also contain potassium chloride which can be harmful in large amounts, particularly if you have kidney problems or if you are taking medication for heart failure or high blood pressure.

Healthier aging and Longevity

Consume plenty of the following:
- Asparagus
- Avocados
- Beans
- Brewers yeast
- Chicken (lean)
- Citrus fruits
- Fish
- Flaxseeds
- Fruit (deeply colored)
- Garlic
- Red grapes or red grape juice
- Kefir

- Leafy greens
- Oats
- Onions
- Pomegranates
- Raw vegetables
- Red peppers
- Sauerkraut
- Strawberries
- Soy products
- Tomatoes
- Turkey
- Water (drink a glass every two waking hours)
- Wheat germ
- Whole grains
- Red wine (occasionally)
- Yogurt

To fight aging – Detoxify

Apples

Help to correct skin and liver disorders. It has a laxative effect, and is a valuable aid to digestion and weight loss.

Beet juice

Nourishes the liver. The liver is one of the most important organs of the body, as it has hundreds of different functions. If our liver is functioning well, most likely everything else in your body is too.

Cabbage

It is excellent for alleviating stomach ailments, especially when combined with comfrey. It's high in vitamin K and cancer-fighting indoles.

Carrot juice

Is high in antioxidants, including beta-carotene and vitamins A, C, and E. It is filled with minerals and anti-aging enzymes. One caveat on carrot juice, since it is high in natural sugar, this juice should be diluted with water, especially if you have a blood sugar imbalance.

Celery

Is moderately high in sodium, not the bad-for-you salt shaker kind, but the good, natural kind that promotes good cell chemistry.

Melon juices

Are wonderful kidney cleansers. The rind provides a wide range of enzymes, minerals, and chlorophyll. Drink melon juice alone, not in combination with other fruits or vegetables.

Pineapple juice

Contains bromelain, which has an anti-inflammatory effect. This is especially good for alleviating arthritic symptoms.

Red Grapes

The skins of red grapes reduce plaque in the walls of arteries.

Longevity

Eat chocolate and whole wheat bread

Athlete's Foot

Soak your feet in a basin of warm water with a few crushed garlic cloves and a splash of rubbing alcohol.

Brain Development in Infants

Feed infants lots of:
- Eggs
- Fish
- Flaxseed

Brain and Brain Function

Consume the following:
- Eggs
- Walnuts
- Wine

Bruising

When bruising appears for no apparent reason, the cause may be your diet rather than your clumsiness. A vitamin deficiency can sometimes cause unexplained bruising. Keep up your vitamin K and get your fill of vitamin C.

Burns

For little kitchen burns, run cold water over them, then apply a slice of Onion to block the pain receptors. Onion juices have antibacterial properties that may help prevent infection.

Another way to help relieve pain from a burn is to rub Garlic Oil onto a burn.

Calluses

Eat pineapple

Cells and Cellular Repair

Eat plenty of the following:
- Garlic
- Onions
- Grapefruit

Cramps and Pain Management

Menstrual Cramps

Supplement your diet with omega-3 fatty acids to make yoru menstrual cycles more regular.

Premenstrual Syndrome (P. M. S.)

Consume the following:
- Bananas
- Cheese
- Milk
- Pasta
- Whole Wheat Bread

Menstrual Pain and Regularity

Eat plenty of the following:
- Fish with Omega-3 Fatty Acids...
- Alaska king crab
- Atlantic mackerel
- Bluefish
- European anchovy
- Lake trout
- Northern lobster
- Pink salmon
- Pacific oysters

- Sardines in sardine oil
- Scallops
- Shrimp
- Striped bass
- Swordfish
- Tuna

Bloating

Eat Basil.

Leg Cramps

Consume the following:
- Bananas
- Orange Juice
- Sweet Potatoes

Muscle Cramps

Eat cheese

Aching Joints

Relaxing in a warm bath may ease your aching joints, but drinking a glass of cool water may also help. Water helps cushion and lubricate your joints. Eight glasses of water a day will help keep your joints gliding smoothly.

Pain Management

Eat chilies.

Relaxation

Eat Rosemary.

Cuts

Eat Bok Choy and drink wine.

Dehydration

Dehydration is caused by consuming alcohol, caffeine, and salt. Alcohol and caffeine should be cut out completely and your salt intake should be reduced to help prevent dehydration and to help fight or help to prevent kidney stones.

Dizziness

To make your own smelling salts, place 1 to 4 drops of Essential Rosemary Oil on a tissue and wave it under your nose.

Enzyme Activity

Eat Pomegranates.

Exercise Performance

Eat mint.

Fatigue

Eat mint and raisins

Fibroids

Eat spinach

Hair
Dry Hair

To add shine to dull hair, mash a very ripe avocado and massage the pulp into your wet hair for about 5 minutes. Leave in for 10 minutes to an hour, then rinse. It may take several washes to remove it all.

Hair Loss

Eat the following:
- Beans
- Brown rice
- Brewer's yeast
- Fish
- Lean poultry
- Nuts
- Oats

- Vegetables
- Whole grains

Vitamin B promotes hair growth and Iron is essential for hair growth.

Take a spoonful of unsulfured blackstrap molasses every day, and include several of the following foods in you diet:

- Berries
- Cashews
- Dried fruits
- Figs
- Green leafy vegetables (except spinach)
- Leeks

To improve Hair Growth, apply 3 to 5 drops of Rosemary essential oil per 1 ounce of shampoo daily to improve scalp circulation.

Hangnails

Eat Bok Choy.

Hangover

Basil can help reduce the resulting bloating and flatulence. Make a tea by steeping 2 tablespoons of chopped fresh basil leaves or 2 teaspoons of dried leaves in 1 cup of boiled water for about 15 minutes; then strain and sip.

Headaches

Garlic is nature's aspirin, dilating the veins and arteries to relieve congestion. Squeeze some garlic juice into a teaspoon of honey. It's an old American Indian remedy.

Migraine Headaches

The smell of green apples can reduce a migraine headache.

Don't forget your Omega 3's. Eat fish at least 3 times a week.

An herbal footbath can soothe your headache. Mix one teaspoon of powdered mustard or ginger with water as hot as you can stand it in a plastic basin big enough for both feet.

Drape a thick towel across the top to hold in the heat. Lean back, close your eyes, breathe deeply, and relax for about 15 minutes.

Calcium and vitamin D can help relieve migraines in people with low blood levels of vitamin D.

Watch out for the three C's. Cheese, chocolate, and citrus; they can trigger headaches.

Caffeine can cause headaches. If you drink more than 8 oz of caffeine a day, it is best to gradually cut back on the caffeine to avoid headaches.

Place salt in a dry pan and heat until it's very warm but not hot. Wrap the salt in a thin dishtowel. If the headache is in front, press the salt pack to the back of your head and rub. The dry heat will draw the pain away from where it's hurting.

Headaches may signal heart disease if they begin during exercise then go away when you rest. It's possible that an undetected chest pain travels along nerves from the heart to the head where it is more noticeable, or the diseased heart causes more pressure in the head because of poor circulation.

This type of cardiac headache may occur in people whose headaches begin after the age of 50, who are at risk of heart disease due to high blood pressure, diabetes, smoking, or family history.

Metabolism

Increase your metabolism by eating mushrooms

Energy

Increase your energy by eating the following:

- Bananas
- Beans
- Beef
- Chicken
- Pasta
- Peas
- Potatoes
- Prunes
- Raisins
- Turkey
- Watermelon

Hiccups

Eat a papaya

Hot Flashes

Consume soy

Hydration

Eat the following:
- Celery
- Cucumbers
- Watermelon

Immune System

To improve your Immune System, eat the following:
- Asparagus
- Beef
- Broccoli sprouts

- Brussels sprouts
- Canola Oil
- Cantaloupe
- Chicken
- Chives
- Curry Powder
- Eggs
- Garlic
- Kiwifruit
- Lettuce
- Mushrooms
- Nectarines
- Okra
- Oranges
- Papaya
- Peaches
- Pineapple
- Pork
- Pumpkin
- Quinoa
- Seeds (Pumpkin, Sesame, Sunflower)
- Shellfish

- Squash
- Sweet Potatoes
- Tea
- Turkey
- Yogurt

Infections

To fight infections, consume the following:
- Basil
- Ginger
- Onions
- Turkey
- Wine

Yeast Infections

To stop a yeast infection, eat sweet potatoes and yogurt.

Inflammation

To reduce inflammation, eat the following:
- Basil

- Fennel
- Ginger

Too much acid in the food causes inflammation, which causes pain.

Lactose Intolerance

Try adding a few teaspoons of cocoa to your milk.

Dry, Brittle Nails

Soak your hands in ½ cup of warm olive oil for 15 to 30 minutes.

Nerve Health

B vitamins are healing for the nerves, especially optic nerves. Eat lots of garlic.

Wound Healing

Consume the following:
- Bok Choy
- Horseradish
- Lettuce
- Oranges
- Papaya
- Peaches
- Potatoes
- Strawberries

Wrinkles

To reduce or prevent wrinkles, eat the following:
- Blueberries
- Oranges
- Rosemary

Miscellaneous Tips:

- Safe Red Dye

Use beet juice instead of artificial food coloring. Unlike some synthetic dyes, beet juice is safe, because it does not trigger liver cancer cell growth.

- Toast Sesame Seeds

Place a nonstick skillet over a high heat and sprinkle in a tablespoon or two of sesame seeds. As the pan heats up, the seeds will begin to pop like popcorn. Shake the pan as you would if you were popping popcorn the old fashioned way. Shake until they are golden brown; sprinkle over salads, cooked veggies, Asian stir-fries, or broiled chicken, fish, or shrimp.

- Your body needs Vitamin C to absorb iron. Eat citrus fruit after an iron-rich meal.

- It is best to take calcium supplements between meals, because some foods contain substances which may compete with calcium for absorption in your body.

- Blueberries contain more antioxidants than any other fruit. They have anti inflammatory effects, improve mental

106

performance and also reduce the rates of urinary-tract infection. Healthful cousins include red grapes, cranberries, blackberries, cherries, raspberries, boysenberries, and strawberries. Eat one to two cups fresh or frozen daily.

• Spinach is rich in the antioxidants lutein and beta-carotene. Healthful cousins include kale, collards, swiss chard, mustard greens, and Romaine lettuce. Your goal is to eat two cups raw or one cup steamed every day.

• Oats are a rich source of fiber including beta-glucans, which help to protect against heart disease. Oats also have minerals, including magnesium, potassium, zinc, copper, manganese and selenium, all of which lower the risk of high blood pressure, diabetes, cancer, and heart disease. Healthful cousins include wheat germ, flaxseed, whole wheat, barley, buckwheat, millet, and amaranth. Five to seven daily servings is recommended.

• Pumpkin is rich in carotenoids, it is also the best source of the combination of alpha-carotene (twice as much as carrots) and beta-carotene – which work optimally as a team.

Carotenoid-rich foods (not supplements) have been shown to reduce the risk for lung, colon, breast, and skin cancers. Canned 100% pure pumpkin is just as nutritious as fresh. Healthful cousins include carrots, sweet potatoes, and butternut squash. You need to eat ½ cup most days.

• Tomatoes have been linked to reduced rates of cancer, particularly prostate malignancies. When joined with lutein, lycopene also fights age-related mascular degeneration. Cooked tomatoes are most readily absorbed by the body. Healthful cousins include watermelon and pink grapefruit. Your goal is to eat one daily serving of processed tomatoes or 1/2 cup of sauce, or one watermelon wedge, ½ pink grapefruit, and multiple servings of fresh tomatoes each week.

• Walnuts contain omega-3 fatty acids, vitamin E, potassium, protein, fiber, and cholesterol-lowering compounds known as plant sterols. Studies suggest that eating about one ounce, about a handful, of nuts five times a week lowers the risk for heart attack by up to 50%. Beware, nuts are high in calories, so do not overindulge. Healthful cousins include almonds, pistachios, sesame seeds, and pecans.

- Try to incorporate oranges, soy, tea (black or green), raw or cooked broccoli, yogurt with live cultures, skinless turkey, and/or beans (Pinto, Navy, Lima, or Chickpeas) in your diet on all or most days of the week.

- Protein is vital to maintaining all the cells, muscles, and other tissues of the body.

- Fiber aids in digestion and reduces cholesterol.

- Water adds volume without calories. Foods with high water content fill you up just as effectively as those that are loaded with fats and sugars. To add more water to your daily diet, start your meals with soup whenever possible, steam vegetables rather than baking or grilling them as this will keep their water content high and eat water-rich stew as a main dish.

- Eat frequent meals. Six small meals and snacks a day will keep your energy level up and your hunger down.

- Buy only salmon that is specifically marked wild Alaskan. You should try to eat three ounces of fish, two to four times per week. Healthful cousins include Halibut, Sardines with the bones, Herring, Sea Bass and Trout, which are low in mercury. Canned albacore tuna is rich in omega-3's but it's best to limit consumption to one can per week because of possible mercury content.

- British researchers from the Southampton University have found that boys born with a low birth weight are more likely to have an increased risk of heart disease later in life.

Eight year olds who were smaller at birth are more likely to have vascular resistance, a property of blood vessels that makes it harder for the blood to be pumped though. Even though this vascular resistance does not cause an immediate problem for a child, there is some suggestion that it might increase the chance of blood pressure problems in adulthood.

No such problem was seen in girls who were born with a low birth weight.

Earlier studies have linked heart disease and diabetes to low birth weight.

Body Food

Check out the amazing clues that food hold for us.

• A sliced carrot looks like the pupil, iris and radiating lines of the human eye. And eating carrots greatly enhances the blood flow to and function of the eyes.

• A Tomato has four chambers and is red. The heart has four chambers and is red. Research shows tomatoes are loaded with lycopine and are indeed pure heart and blood food.

• Grapes hang in a cluster that has the shape of the heart. Each grape looks like a blood cell and research shows grapes are also profound heart and blood vitalizing food.

• A Walnut looks like a little brain, a left and right hemisphere, upper cerebrums and lower cerebellums. Even the wrinkles or folds on the nut are just like the neo-cortex. We now know walnuts help develop more than three (3) dozen neuron-transmitters for brain function.

• Kidney Beans actually heal and help maintain kidney function and yes, they look exactly like the human kidneys.

- Celery, Bok Choy, Rhubarb, and many more look just like bones. These foods specifically target bone strength. Bones are 23% sodium and these foods are 23% sodium. If you don't have enough sodium in your diet, the body pulls it from the bones, thus making them weak. These foods replenish the skeletal needs of the body.

- Sweet Potatoes look like the pancreas and actually balance the glycemic index of diabetics.

- Avocadoes, Eggplant, and Pears target the health and function of the womb and cervix of the female and they look just like these organs. Research shows that when a woman eats one avocado a week, it balances hormones, sheds unwanted birth weight, and prevents cervical cancers. And how profound is this? It takes exactly nine months to grow an avocado from blossom to ripened fruit. There are over 14,000 photolytic chemical constituents of nutrition in each one of these foods (modern science has only studied and named about 141 of them.

- Male fertility can be maintained by eating bananas, figs, and olives.

- Bananas help to increase fertility, and cure impotency.

- Figs are full of seeds and hang in twos when they grow. Figs increase the mobility of male sperm and increase the number of sperm as well as overcome male sterility.

- Olives help to ensure fertility as well as sexual potency in men.

- Olives, which resemble ovaries, assist the health and function of the ovaries.

- Oranges, grapefruits, and other citrus fruits look just like the mammary glands of the female and actually assist the health of the breasts and the movement of lymph in and out of the breasts.

- Onions look like the body's cells. Research shows onions help clear waste materials from all of the body cells. They even produce tears which wash the epithelial layers of the eyes. A working companion, garlic, also helps eliminate waste materials and dangerous free radicals from the body.

REFERENCES

AARP The Magazine September/October 2008

A Jerry Baker Health Book Giant Book of Kitchen Counter Cures By: Karen Cicero and Colleen Pierre, M.S., R.D.

Bottom Line's Presscription for Natural Cures By: James F. Balch, MD and Mark Stengler, ND

Bottom Line Year Book 2006

God's Pharmacy

Maude Grieve 1931 Herb book, a Modern Herbal

MayoClinic.com

Miracle Medicine Foods By: Rex Adams

Nature's Prescriptions

Thaindian News

The Complete Encyclopedia of Natural Healing By: Gary Null, Ph.D.

The Healing Garden 1994 at Michael Bell and Kangaroo Press.

Printed by Libri Plureos GmbH in Hamburg,
Germany